BOOK DESCRIPTION

With so many deaths each year from around the world, it has been related to poor health choices we make, and certain lifestyles. Many people tend to avoid the topic of death. Death is an inevitable event that we all must come to terms with, especially those who are serious about their spiritual development.

The phenomenon called death is the end of everything that you may know. Your body, mind, work, purposes, the things that you have built up, the things that you want to do, the things that you are yet to complete – there is an end to all these when death appears. That is the fact: the complete end.

For some persons, death isn't a source of fear or uncertainty, instead, it is a doorway, an integral part of existence and also an opportunity to elevate our consciousness. There is an ancient teaching that says if we want to know what happens when we die, we must look to what happens when we sleep at night. 20 per cent to 40 per cent of deaths from each cause could be prevented, according to a study from the Centers for Disease Control and Prevention. So how can you then avoid an early death?

It was once thought that lifespan was mostly determined by our genetics. While having good genes plays a major role, your genes may only be responsible for about 20% of how long you live. The rest largely depends on the secret findings revealed in this book.

This book attempts to alert the readers to certain ways to avoid death. Several chapters describe some major threats that are likely to kill people, ways to prevent death and secret foods that can help keep you healthy and make you live longer too.

This short book nominally explores the common ways to avoid death in the modern era. It's conciseness gives straight to the point approaches you'll need to live longer. It's better to read a short book that makes you live longer than read a long book full of BS, and nothing to gain.

Brief Contents

How to Avoid Death

Discover the secret foods that can deter

diseases and make you live you longer

Dedication

This book is dedicated to every survivor out there who is making the most of life and wish to live more of it.

Preface

Death is considered an intrinsic part of life. Talking about the likely outcomes of illness is a very important part of health care. Health professionals and patients vary in the language they use and in their comfort regarding such topics. Individuals also vary in their comfort level regarding the amount of information and involvement in decision-making that they want. Very sick patients and their loved ones should try to understand the likely future course of their illness, as well as the options for living with any disabilities and family situations.

A dying process that gives an individual choice about treatment, saying your last goodbye, and also taking care of final arrangements is what many people secretly hope for. Such a death can be considered a "good death". Sadly, many deaths do not occur this way. Most deaths do not include such a dialogue session with family members or being able to die in familiar surroundings. People usually die suddenly and alone, people leave their homes and never get to return. Wives precede husbands in death, children precede parents, and the homeless are bereaved by total strangers or nobody at all.

CHAPTER 1

Whether we want to acknowledge it or not, many people fear death. Death remains a great mystery, one of the main issues with which religion, philosophy and science have wrestled since the beginning of human history. Although dying is a natural existence, many cultures find it unique in the extent to which death is viewed as a taboo topic. Rather than discussing it, we incline to view death as a feared opponent that should be defeated with modern-day medicine and machines.

Can we fully know and comprehend the full meaning of death? That is, can the mind be fully trifle, with no remnant of the past? Whether that is logical or not is something we can explore, search out diligently, actively, and work hard to find out. But if the mind barely holds to what it calls living, which is suffering, this entire process of accumulation, and tries to resist the other, then it knows neither life nor death. So the issue is to free the mind from the known, from all the things it has gathered, obtained, and experienced so that it is made honourable and can therefore appreciate that which is death, the unknowable.

Death is the total termination of life processes that eventually occurs in all living organisms. The state of human death has always been concealed by mystery and superstitions, and its exact definition remains very controversial. The meaning differs according to culture and legal systems. Before the 20th century, death was greatly eschewed in serious scientific, and philosophical assumptions. It was disregarded in biological research, and being beyond the physician's ministrations, was considered insignificant by medical practice. In modern times, however, the study of death has now become a central concern in all these disciplines and many others.

To discover what death is, there must be no distance between death and you who are existing with your troubles and all the rest of it. You must comprehend the importance of death and live with it while you are somewhat alert, not dead, not quite dead yet. That thing called death is the end of everything that you may know. Your body, mind, work, purposes, the things that you have built up, the things that you want to do, the things that you are yet to complete – there is an end to all these when death appears. That is the fact: the complete end. What happens after is quite another issue; that is not important because you will not be able to ask what happens afterwards if there is no fear. Then death becomes something remarkable, not sadistically, not abnormally or unhealthily, because death then is something uncommon, and there is great beauty in that which is not known.

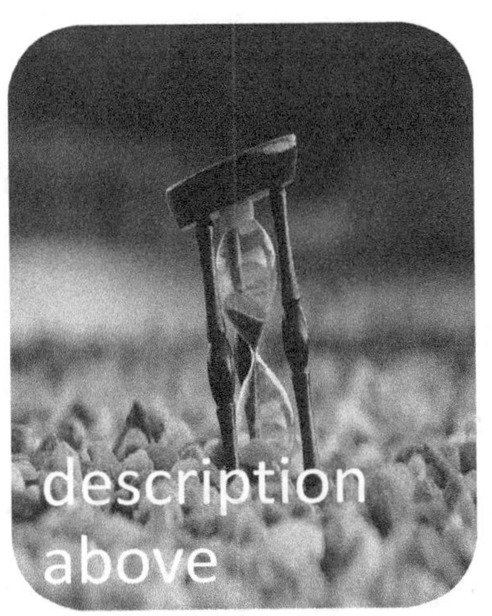
description
above

The statistics

With so many deaths each year from around the world, it has been related to poor health choices we make, and certain lifestyles. World health leaders have set a goal of reducing the number of preventable deaths by 25% from 2010 rates by 2025. That would save over 37 million lives over 15 years. Everyone wants to live as long as possible, without substantial pain or disability. Americans are now living longer than ever, with an expectancy of 78.8 years with both males and females inclusive which ranks 26th in the world when compared to other countries. In America, women tend to live almost five years longer than men. The most common cause of premature death in the U.S., by a vast margin, is cardiovascular disease which includes: heart attack, stroke, lung disease, followed by cancer, and then accidents that lead to deadly injuries.

Death isn't anything most people enjoy thinking about, but at some point, we all reach the end of life, but certain lifestyle choices can help prevent death. The average lifespan in the United States is 75 years old and anyone who dies before 75 is considered to have died prematurely. 20 per cent to 40 per cent of deaths from each cause could be prevented, according to a study from the Centers for Disease Control and Prevention. So how can you then avoid an early death?

Premature death

Death is considered premature when it occurs before someone has had the chance to live a full life. Premature death can be due to illness, accidents, or other factors. While death is always disturbing, premature death can be especially tragic because it signifies lost potential. In many cases, premature death can be preventable, which makes it all the more devastating. Death rates are now dropping in developed countries all thanks to advances in medical care, but there is still much work to be done to reduce the number of premature deaths worldwide. It is important to remember that every life lost to premature death is considered a tragedy that should be avoided if at all possible.

Actual death at some point is not avoidable, but it is possible to increase longevity, which should be enough to allow you to live enough time until you are tired of living at some point. I would estimate that at the end of this century, life expectancy in most developed countries would easily exceed 100 years. Early death for people around the world is most commonly due to illnesses caused by smoking, high blood pressure, high blood cholesterol, alcohol misuse, obesity and physical inactivity.

Lifestyle adjustments on risk factors can help to prevent many diseases. A risk factor is something that makes it more probable that you will acquire a particular disease or medical condition. Some risk factors, such as age, sex and family history, are beyond anybody's control. However, several lifestyle-related risk factors are very much in your control. You can drastically reduce your risk of illness and early death by making a few simple lifestyle adjustments. Risk factors that can be altered include weight, blood pressure and cholesterol level.

The social determinants

The social determinants of health point to key areas in our lives that influence our life, quality, and untimely death. Our lives are not just influenced by science, it is also influenced by the social determinants of health. The social determinants of health are considered to be the factors in which we live, work, and play. They include things like our income, education, housing, and access to healthcare services. Several research has shown that the social determinants of health play a very crucial role in our life expectancy. This is because poverty can lead to poor nutrition, stress, and unhealthy behaviours. It can also make it very difficult to access good healthcare. By appreciating the social determinants of health, we can take steps to reduce our chances of premature death.

CHAPTER 2

WHY DO PEOPLE DIE?

The leading reason for human death in most developing countries is an infectious disease. One of the leading causes in developed countries is atherosclerosis which leads to heart disease and stroke, cancer, and other diseases related to obesity and ageing. By a very wide margin, the largest unifying cause of death in the developed world is biological ageing, which leads to various complications known as ageing-associated diseases. These conditions result in loss of homeostasis and cardiac arrest which leads to loss of oxygen and nutrient supply, causing the irreversible breakdown of the brain and other important body tissues. Roughly 150,000 people die each day across the globe, and about two-thirds die of age-related causes.

With enhanced medical capability, dying has now become a condition to be managed. Home deaths, once commonplace, are now unusual in the developed world. Many leading causes of death in developed countries can be discontinued by diet and physical activity, but the accelerating incidence of disease with age still puts limits on human longevity. The evolutionary cause of ageing is only just beginning to be comprehended. It has been proposed that direct intervention in the ageing process may now be the most effective intervention against major causes of death.

It is very important to understand the cause of death and the risk factor associated with premature death. Every death is attributed to a single underlying cause, the cause that resulted in the series of events leading to death. This is quite different from the deaths that occurred due to certain risk factors. These deaths are an estimation of the decrease of the number of deaths that would be achieved if the risk factors to which a population is exposed would be eradicated, in the case of tobacco smoking, for example, or reduced to an optimal, healthy level, in the case of the body-mass index.

In medicine, statistics and law, the reason for death is an official determination of conditions that leads to human death, which may be recorded on a death certificate. The reason for death is deduced by a medical examiner. The reason for death is a specific disease or injury, in contrast to the manner of death which is a small number of categories like natural, accident, suicide, and homicide, which have different legal implications.

Health departments have discouraged classifying old age as one of the causes of death because doing so has no benefit to public health or medical research. Ageing is not a scientifically acknowledged cause of death; It is supposed that there is always a more direct cause, although it may be unknown in certain cases and could be one of several ageing-associated diseases. As an indirect or non-determinative factor, biological ageing is one of the biggest contributors to deaths worldwide.

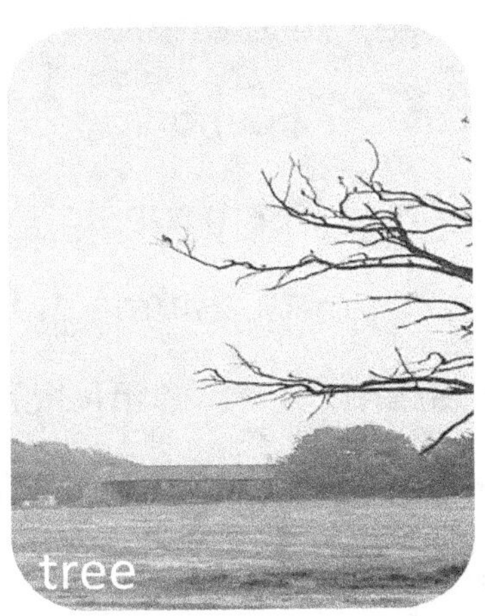

The top causes of death worldwide, in order of the total number of lives lost, are associated with these three broad topics: cardiovascular which includes: ischaemic heart disease, stroke; respiratory conditions including chronic obstructive pulmonary disease, lower respiratory infections; and neonatal conditions which include birth asphyxia, birth trauma, neonatal sepsis and infections, and preterm birth complications. Causes of death can be grouped into three categories: communicable, which could be infectious and parasitic diseases and maternal, perinatal and nutritional conditions; non-communicable (chronic); and injuries.

The world's biggest killer is ischaemic heart disease, which is responsible for 16% of the world's total deaths. Chronic obstructive pulmonary disease (COPD) and stroke are the 2nd and 3rd leading causes of death.

Lower respiratory tract infections have remained the world's most deadly communicable disease, it is ranked as the 4th leading cause of death.

However, the number of deaths has gone down substantially: in 2019 it claimed over 2.6 million lives, 460 000 fewer than in 2000. Neonatal conditions are ranked 5th. Deaths from different neonatal conditions are one of the categories for which the global decrease in deaths in absolute numbers over the past two decades has been the greatest. Certain noncommunicable diseases that lead to death are on the rise. Trachea, bronchus and lung cancer deaths have risen from 1.2 million to 1.8 million and are now ranked 6th among the leading causes of death.

In 2019, Alzheimer's disease and other types of dementia are ranked as the 7th leading cause of death. Females are disproportionately affected. Globally, 65 per cent of deaths from Alzheimer's and other forms of dementia are females. One of the largest deteriorations in the number of deaths is from diarrhoeal diseases, with global deaths falling from 2.6 million in 2000 to 1.5 million in 2019. Diabetes has recently entered the top 10 causes of death, following a significant percentage increase of 70% since 2000. Diabetes is also accountable for the largest rise in male deaths among the top 10, with an 80% increase since 2000.

Several diseases which were among the top 10 causes of death in 2000 are no longer on the list. HIV/AIDS is one of them. Deaths from HIV/AIDS have fallen by 51% during the last 25 years, moving from the world's 8th leading cause of death in 2000 to the 19th. Kidney diseases have risen greatly around the world. The mortality rate is rapidly increasing.

People living in a low-income country are more likely to die of a communicable disease than a non-communicable disease. Although there is a global decline, six of the top 10 causes of death in low-income countries are communicable diseases.

Malaria, tuberculosis and HIV/AIDS remain in the top 10. However, the three are declining significantly. The largest decline among the top 10 deaths in this group has been for HIV/AIDS, with 59% fewer deaths than in 2000. Diarrhoeal diseases are also an important cause of death in low-income countries: they rank in the top 5 causes of death for this income category. Diarrhoeal diseases are declining in certain low-income countries, representing the second biggest decrease. Deaths due to chronic obstructive pulmonary disease are particularly rare in low-income countries compared to other income groups.

It is crucial to know why people die to improve how people live. Measuring how many people die each year assists to assess the effectiveness of our health systems and directing resources to where they are needed most. For example, mortality data can assist the government focus on activities and resource allocation among sectors such as transportation, food and agriculture, and the environment as well as health. COVID-19 highlighted the importance for countries to invest in civil registration and vital statistics systems to enable daily counting of deaths, and direct prevention and treatment efforts. It has also disclosed intrinsic fragmentation in data collection systems in most low-income countries, where policymakers still do not know with confidence how many people die and for what causes.

World Health Organization has developed standards and best practices for data collection, processing and synthesis through the compact and improved International Classification of Diseases (ICD-11) – a digital platform that enables reporting of timely and accurate data for causes of death for countries to routinely generate and use health information that conforms to international standards.

The regular compilation and estimation of high-quality data on deaths and causes of death, as well as data on disability, disaggregated by age, sex and geographic location, is fundamental for enhancing health and decreasing deaths and disability in the world.

Death is something no one can completely avoid. It is the one certainty in life. However, death can come sooner than it should if we engage in dangerous behaviours. By understanding what those behaviours are and how to avoid them, we can all help to reduce the risk of premature death. Many factors can contribute to premature death.

To quickly summarise this, here are a few reasons why people die:

- ★ Illnesses, which could be acquired or due to genetics
- ★ Accidents
- ★ Suicide
- ★ Homicide
- ★ Ageing
- ★ Poor lifestyle habits.

CHAPTER 3

With so many deaths each year from around the world directly related to poor health choices we make, world health leaders around the world have set a goal of lowering preventable deaths by 25 per cent by 2025. This will save 37 million lives over 15 years. Although death is not predictable, there are some lifestyle changes and activities that can help prevent death to an extent, these include:

1) Be more physically active.

A very important factor in decreasing your risk of dying prematurely from cardiovascular disease is exercising regularly and maintaining a healthy weight. Obesity puts lots of stress on the heart and blood vessels, which leads to dysfunction eventually. Just 30 minutes of mild-to-moderate cardiovascular exercise every day is linked to better health and longevity, exercising can reduce blood pressure and cholesterol levels, as well as reduce weight. You can start with walking around your neighbourhood, if weather permits you, then change to more difficult terrain, treadmills and/or cycling.

Avoid vigorous exercise when starting, especially if you have a known heart condition. Vigorous exercise such as marathon running can temporarily increase your blood pressure and strain on the heart, which may trigger a heart attack. Only thirty minutes of daily exercise is good for your health and an hour is even better, but much beyond that amount isn't proven to be significantly more beneficial. Types of moderate-intensity exercise can include ballroom dancing, biking slowly, using your manual wheelchair, walking, and water aerobics. Extremely strenuous activities are biking up hills, basketball, swimming laps, and marathon running.

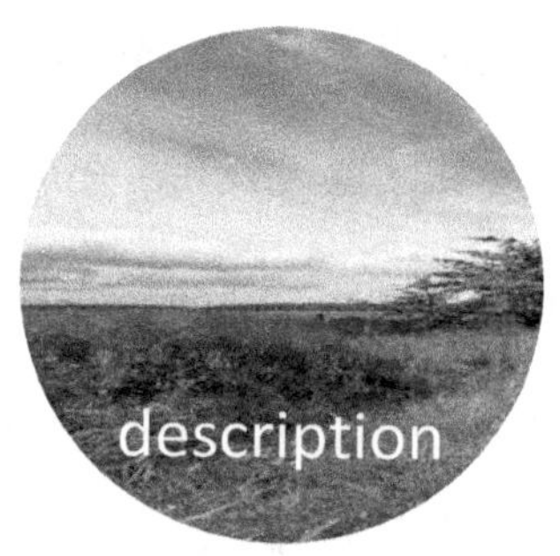

2) Avoid smoking.

Smoking tobacco is a very harmful habit you can do regularly. It is well established that smoking can damage nearly every organ of the body and causes many diseases, including all sorts of cardiovascular-related problems, which contribute considerably to premature death. Smoking is assessed to increase your risk of coronary heart disease and stroke due to atherosclerosis by up to 4 times compared to people who do not smoke at all. Cigarettes contain different toxic compounds that can damage your blood vessels and other body tissues.

Cigarette smoking causes an average of 480,000 deaths each year in the United States, which is about one in every five deaths. Smoking is also considered the leading cause of chronic obstructive pulmonary disease of the lungs and lung cancer. You can make use of nicotine patches or gum to help wean yourself off cigarettes.

description

3) Maintain healthy cholesterol levels.

Eating fat, even saturated fat, can be healthy in moderation, after all, fatty acids are required to make all cell membranes in the body, but too much "bad fat" can affect cardiovascular health. Although saturated fat, which is the kind found in animal products is often considered unhealthy, the kind that causes problems is trans fat. Trans fats raise the bad LDL cholesterol and lower the good HDL cholesterol in the blood, which increases the risk of having a heart attack and stroke.

The normal total cholesterol levels in the blood should be less than 200 mg/dL. LDL cholesterol should be less than 100 mg/dL, while HDL levels should be above 60 mg/dL for total protection against cardiovascular disease. The healthiest fats are considered to be monounsaturated and polyunsaturated plant-based fats. Foods that are rich in polyunsaturated fat include safflower, sesame and sunflower seeds, corn oil and soybeans; whereas great sources of monounsaturated fat include avocados, canola, olive and peanut oils.

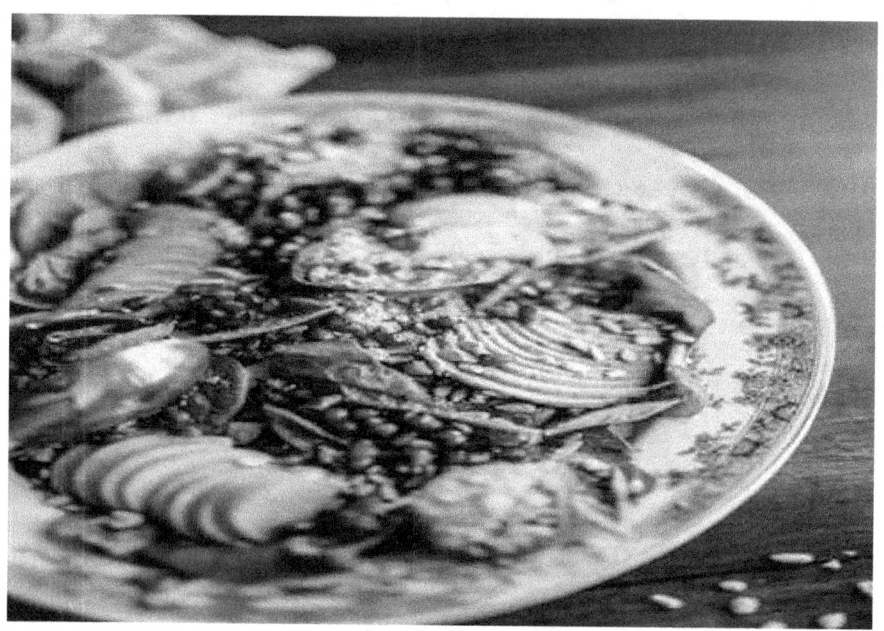

4) Control your blood pressure.

High blood pressure often called hypertension is often referred to as a silent killer because it doesn't often cause obvious symptoms until it's too late. High blood pressure strains the heart and damages the insides of arteries over time. It promotes atherosclerosis, also stroke and kidney disease. Blood pressure can be effectively reduced with medication, although some people experience significant side effects from these medications. Natural ways of reducing blood pressure include losing excess weight, eating a healthy diet based on lots of fresh produce, cutting back on salt consumption, regular exercise and controlling your stress level, breathing techniques, and yoga.

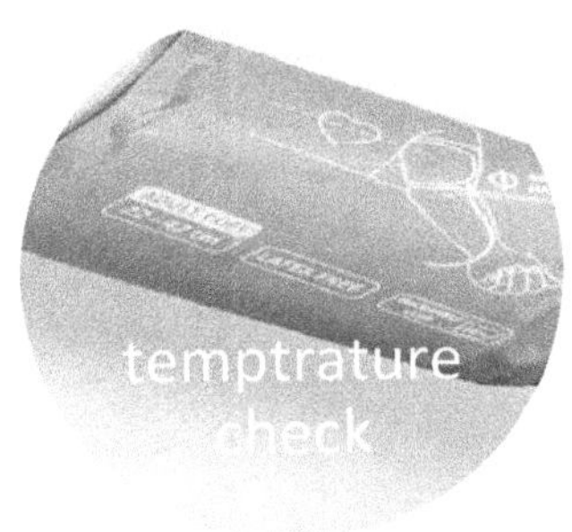

5) Reduce your alcohol consumption.

Based on recent research, there is a strong linkage between drinking alcohol and several types of cancer, especially cancer of the mouth, throat, breast, liver and large intestine. Ethanol, the type of alcohol commonly taken, is a well-known human carcinogen. The more alcohol a person consumes regularly over time, the higher the risk of developing cancer and dying premature death. As such, either you completely stop drinking alcohol or you limit your consumption to no more than one alcoholic beverage in 24 hours. Alcohol is known to thin the blood, which can help lessen the risk of atherosclerosis, but the net impact of ethanol on health is negative.

6) Eat food that contains more antioxidants and fewer preservatives.

Antioxidants are defined as compounds, mostly from plants, fruits and veggies that deter or even stop the oxidation of other molecules in the body. While oxygen is needed in the body, oxidation of certain compounds sometimes becomes a bad thing because it produces free radicals, which can damage the surrounding tissue and even alter its DNA. Free radicals are often linked to cancer, cardiovascular disease and also premature ageing. Preservatives, which are found in most prepared foods, are also damaging to the body due to free radical formation and general toxicity. As such, focusing on consuming antioxidants is a good strategy to prevent cancer.

Compounds that act as strong antioxidants include vitamins C and E, beta-carotene, glutathione, coenzyme Q10, lipoic acid, flavonoids and phenols, among many others. Foods extremely rich in antioxidants include dark-coloured berries, strawberries, apples, cherries, kidney beans and pinto beans. Other foods that are protective against cancer include broccoli, tomatoes, walnuts and garlic.

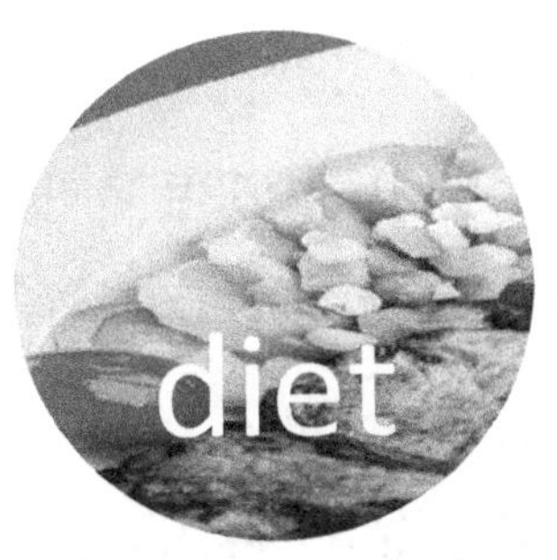

7) Reduce sun exposure.

Sun exposure is needed for life to thrive, but when it becomes excessive especially if you're constantly getting sunburned dramatically heightens the risk of skin cancer. In slightly moderate amounts, especially during the summer months, sunlight triggers vitamin D production in the skin, which has many known benefits including stimulating your immunity and regulating mood. However, the ultraviolet radiation in sunlight can damage skin cells, sometimes even on a DNA level, which leads to mutation of cells and cancer development. Nonetheless, don't avoid the sun, but limit your direct exposure to no more than an hour every day. If you plan on being outside longer, try to cover up with a hat and lightweight breathable cotton clothes, or use natural forms of sunblock and sunscreen.

Skin cancer is one of the most common types of cancer, accounting for about 3.5 million cases a year in the U.S. Basal and squamous cell skin cancers are the most common, but melanoma is more deadly. The major risk factors for skin cancer include pale skin, severe sunburns, older age and weakened immune systems. Also, chronic exposure to coal tar, paraffin, and most hydrocarbon-based products commonly cause skin cancer.

8) Wear your seat belt.

Deadly accidents are another common cause of premature death. Although modern airbags are a great safety feature and can contribute to saving lives, seat belts are still considered a very essential injury prevention tool because they prevent people from being thrown from their vehicles during a crash. It is estimated that seat belt use reduces serious crash-related injuries and deaths by about 50%. As such, always buckle up whenever you enter a vehicle if you want to reduce the risk of premature death from injury. Also, always were a motorcycle helmet to prevent fatal head trauma.

9) Do not drink and drive.

It should be clear that drinking alcohol does not fit with driving a car or operating any heavy equipment. Still, many people keep doing it because alcohol distorts a person's judgement and ability to think clearly. In the United States, an estimated 32% of fatal car accidents involve an intoxicated driver or a pedestrian. In addition to poor judgement, driving intoxicated is very dangerous because alcohol lowers reaction times, decision making and coordination.

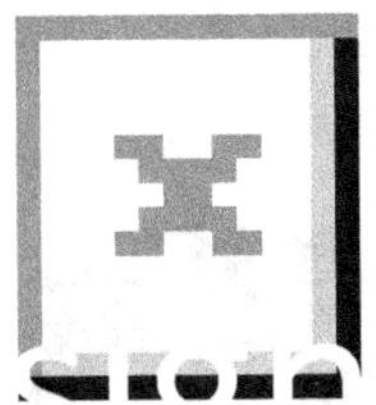

10) Never mix alcohol with drugs.

 Another combination that is unhealthy is drinking alcohol while taking drugs either an illicit prescription or even over-the-counter drugs. The by-products of alcohol and drugs are metabolized in the liver, and sometimes when certain compounds are mixed, reaction can occur. That can severely injure or completely damage your liver. As little as pain relievers, such as acetaminophen, mixed with a glass of wine can lead to liver failure. In addition, taking alcohol with drugs often leads to changes in perception, behaviour, mood, breathing rate, and blood pressure. This can all increase the risk of dying prematurely. Therefore, never combine the two at the same time.

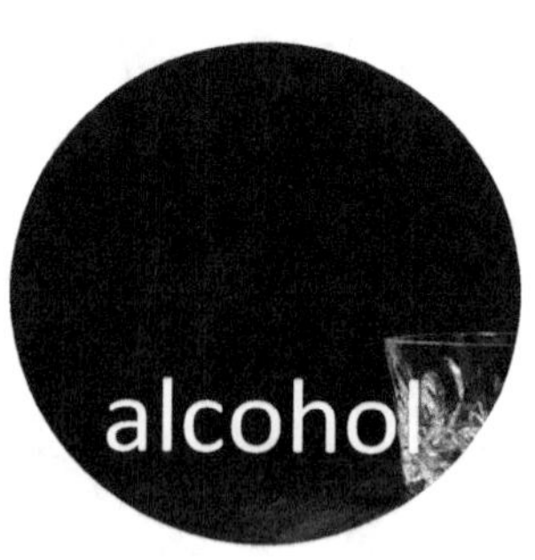

11) Know your family history.

Knowing your family history can give you insight into what might be lurking in your genes, and can potentially help you avoid a death that could have been prevented with mere lifestyle changes or early detection. The dominant causes of death in the United States are heart disease, cancer, and stroke, all of which have genetic components. If you know that heart disease exists in your family, you can make lifestyle changes to reduce your risk, such as eating a healthy diet and exercising regularly. When you know cancer is common in your family, you will consider more frequent screenings. And if a stroke is a problem, you may want to work with your doctor to help manage any underlying conditions, such as high blood pressure.

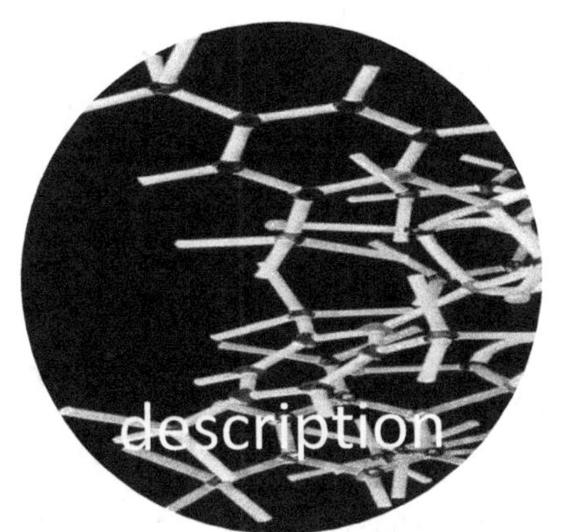

description

12) Always manage your stress levels.

When the body is in an endless fight or flight state, the nervous system can't turn off the stress response. This impacts the heart, digestive and endocrine systems, it messes with our sleep cycle and prevents the body from returning to homeostasis. This results in the development of heart disease, diabetes, autoimmune disorders and neurodegenerative conditions, to name a few. Taking time to relax, implementing a daily breathing or meditation practice and even creating a healthy work/life balance is crucial to lengthening life expectancy.

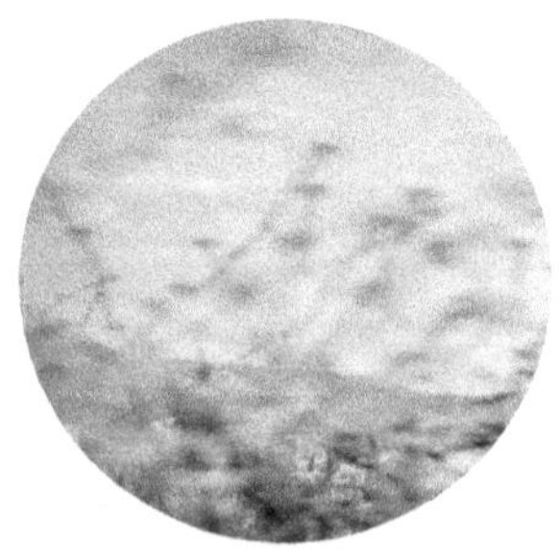

13) Go for routine checkups.

Always ensure that you schedule routine doctor and dental appointments. It is a powerful preventative in the development of life-ending illness. Getting proper lab tests and any other diagnostics that your doctor suggests is very important. Certain screenings such as mammograms, colonoscopies, ultrasounds and scans detect internal abnormalities that may not be causing any physical symptoms yet. This gives you and your doctor time to treat the illness before it is even advanced. In addition to seeing your primary care, dental checkups are also very important. Bacteria in your teeth can lead to a life-threatening infection in your heart valves. Studies have also shown that the state of our oral health can be a sign of other health issues happening within the body.

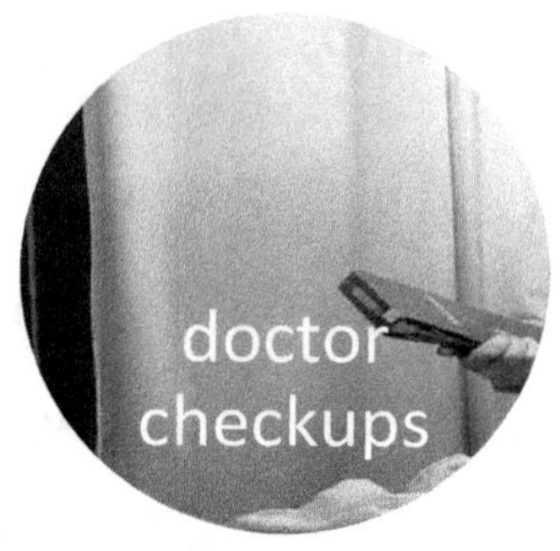

In the next chapter, we'd be looking at secret foods that can increase your life span.

CHAPTER 4

Everyone wishes to live a long and healthy life but what most people don't know is that what you put on your plate can make a huge difference. In addition to following an overall healthy eating pattern, moving your body regularly, and integrating other healthy lifestyle habits can go a long way. It was once thought that lifespan was mostly determined by our genetics. While having good genes plays a major role, your genes may only be responsible for about 20% of how long you live. The rest largely depends on your lifestyle, diet, environment, activity level, social connection, and more. Modern medicine also certainly contributes to longer lifespans, but ageing well isn't just about making it to a certain birthday, it's also about living all of those years to the fullest capacity. These foods below can improve your health and increase longevity.

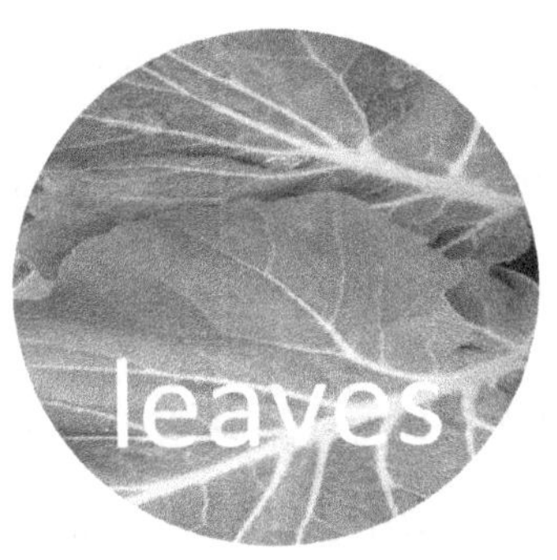

1) Beans

Beans are popular for containing healthy-ageing nutrients. From plant-based proteins to fibre to antioxidants, these little powerhouses have a lot of nutrients. Data shows that eating a plant-based diet is linked to reducing the risk of early death. Swapping out a heavy animal protein with beans a few times a week is a very wise choice to support overall health, says Lauren Manaker, M.S., RDN, LD, Charleston-based dietitian and author of Fueling Male Fertility. Beans contain compounds that are linked to reducing the risk of cancer. Regularly eating beans may also help to reduce the risk of type 2 diabetes, lower cholesterol levels and reduce inflammation. All beans contain important nutrients that can fight off disease and promote longevity. So aim for a variety, but most importantly, choose the ones you will like.

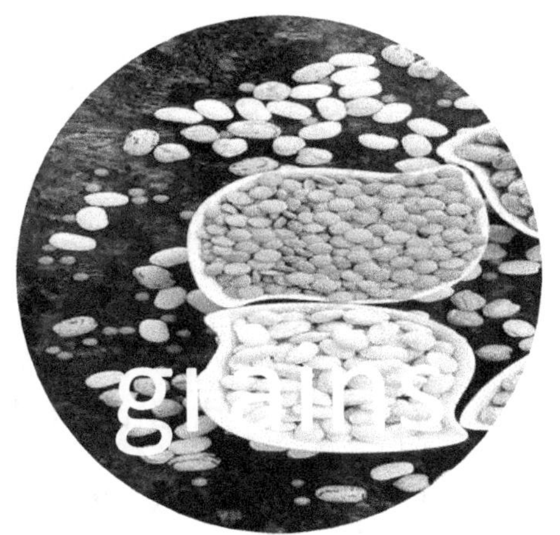

grains

2) Whole grains

Whole grains have been demonized in recent years for their supposed connection to a variety of health concerns. But research now supports the benefits of consuming whole grains for health and longevity. It helps fight cardiovascular disease, dementia and cancer. Consuming three servings of whole grains per day is associated with a 25 per cent lower risk of dying of cardiovascular disease when compared to those that eat fewer than that. Whole grains in their original form such as farro, wheat berries, quinoa, and oats offer the most health benefits, but choosing whole-grain bread and pasta when possible is also suggested. Cornmeal and popcorn are also regarded as whole grains.

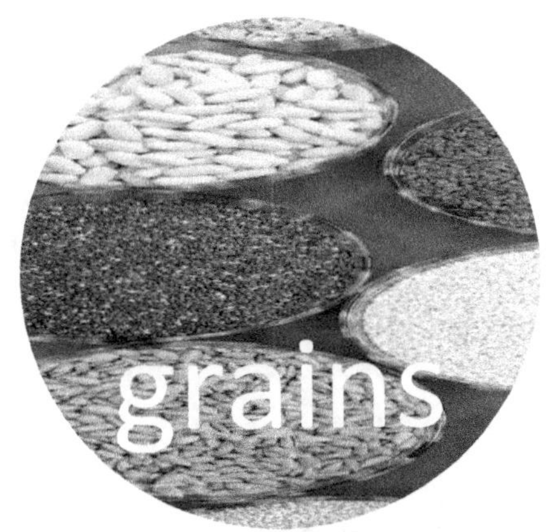
grains

3) Green tea

What's in your mug could be just as important as what's on your plate too. Green tea is popularly known for its potential to reduce cancer risk, but the benefits don't just stop there.

A study looked at green tea consumption and risk of death in those that experienced a stroke or heart attack found that the biggest tea drinkers had up to a 62 per cent lower risk of death when compared to non-green tea drinkers. Green tea contains a very unique polyphenol that has been shown to offer many heart benefits, and likely contributes to this positive benefit of lowering the risk of death.

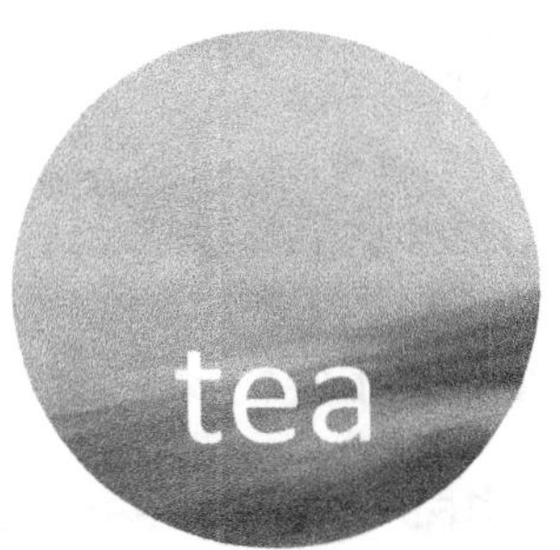
tea

4) Cruciferous Vegetables

Cauliflower, broccoli, brussels sprouts, cabbage, and other cruciferous vegetables are often talked about in their relation to a healthy digestive system which is incredibly important for overall health. But eating these crunchy vegetables is also linked to several benefits related directly to living longer. They are very rich in fibre, antioxidants and vitamins A, C and K. These are associated with healthy ageing. Sulforaphane is an antioxidant primarily found in cruciferous vegetables. It is known to have anticancer benefits, provides possible protection against heart disease, and even supports blood glucose control in people with type 2 diabetes.

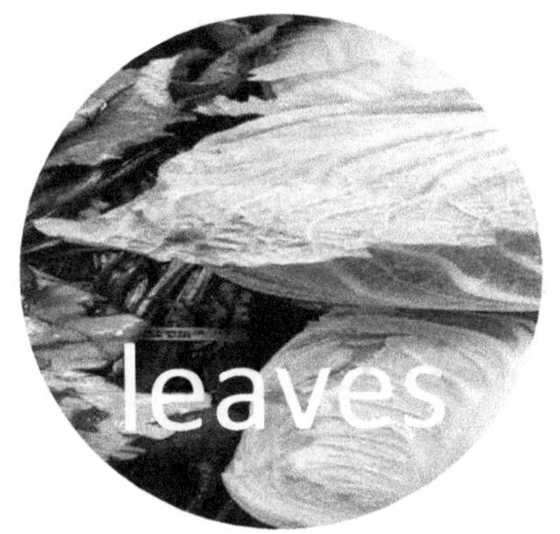
leaves

5) Salmon

Salmon and other fatty fish have vital omega-3 fats, lean protein, B-vitamins, selenium and iron. It offers health benefits such as lowering the risk of heart disease and an 80-90 per cent lower risk of sudden cardiac death. A seafood-rich diet has also been linked to lower the risk of depression and improved memory and cognition. Research has shown that eating just over 2 ounces of fish a day was associated with a 12% reduced risk of dying of all causes. Another large study found a 38% reduced risk of death from Alzheimer's Disease, 20% reduced risk of dying of cancer, and 15-18% reduced risk of death from cardiovascular disease among regular fatty fish eaters.

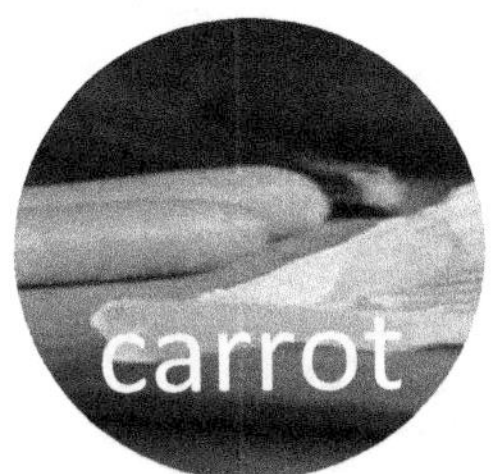
carrot

6) Dark Leafy Greens

Over and over again, data has shown that eating dark leafy greens is linked to a lot of health outcomes, including a reduced risk of early death. An analysis of 13 studies found that regular leafy green consumption was associated with a 15.8% lower risk of developing cardiovascular disease. Other research suggests benefits such as improving mental sharpness and reducing the risk of age-related macular degeneration (AMD). One study that followed 2,800 participants for a period of 15 years found a 35% lower risk of AMD in those that regularly consumed nitrates from vegetables like leafy greens. Dark leafy greens also contain zeaxanthin and lutein, two antioxidants that are healthy for the eye.

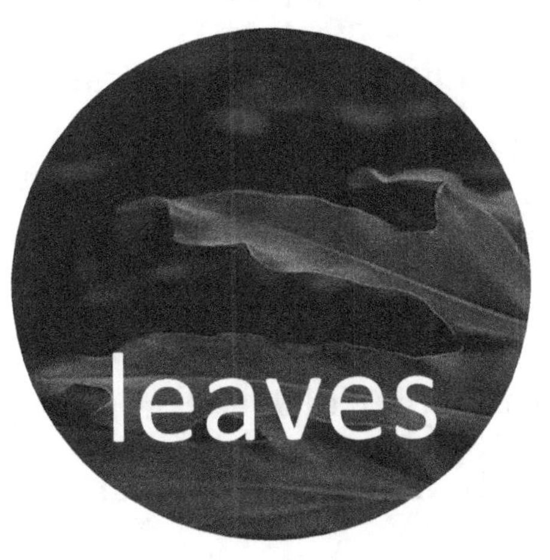
leaves

7) Olive oil

Olive oil is greatly packed with health-promoting compounds. In addition to monounsaturated fats, olive oil also contains polyphenols known for their anti-inflammatory properties, among other benefits. A study evaluating over 7,000 people showed that each 10-gram increase in extra-virgin olive oil consumption per day was linked to a 7% reduced risk of early death. Research has also shown that regular olive oil intake may slow telomere shortening. Telomeres make up the DNA structure and shorter telomeres are a hallmark of ageing. One study that was done among people over the age of 50 found that olive oil consumption improved the successful ageing index. This measured a variety of physical health outcomes such as cardiovascular disease risk factors along with social and mental health outcomes commonly associated with ageing.

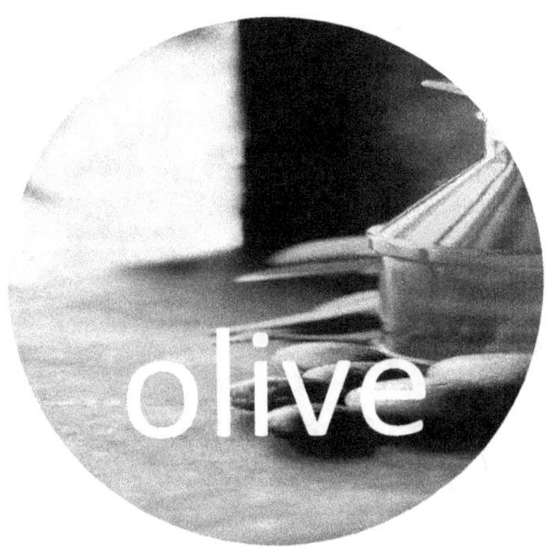

olive

8) Berries

Berries have been studied for health benefits ranging from reducing the risk of cardiovascular disease, protection against cancer, and lower levels of inflammation. What's even more interesting about berries is their potential effect on brain health. The Nurses Health Study, which was made up of over 16,000 participants over the age of 70, found that greater intakes of blueberries and strawberries were linked to slower cognitive decline. Another study showed that blueberry extract improves memory. Whether you prefer strawberries, raspberries, blueberries or blackberries, they all offer health-protective vitamins, minerals, antioxidants and fibre. The antioxidant content in blueberries, raspberries and blackberries also ranks among the highest of all fruits. Berries help to combat free radicals that can cause damage to your cells, as well as inflammation.

9) Walnuts

While all nuts offer great health benefits. Walnuts stand out when it comes to disease prevention and healthy ageing. Eating walnuts is often linked to better heart health, lowering the risk of cancer, reduced inflammation, blood sugar control in people with type 2 diabetes, and better brain health. Regular walnut intake could help you live longer. Researchers have analyzed 18 years of data from the Nurses Health Study and the Health Professionals Follow-Up Study and found that eating at least 5 walnuts per week was attributed with females living longer than males. Experts also believe these benefits come from a combination of the alpha-linoleic acid, omega-3 and certain polyphenols found in walnuts. Polyunsaturated fats, including omega-3s, have also been linked to less joint pain, which improves our quality of life as we age.

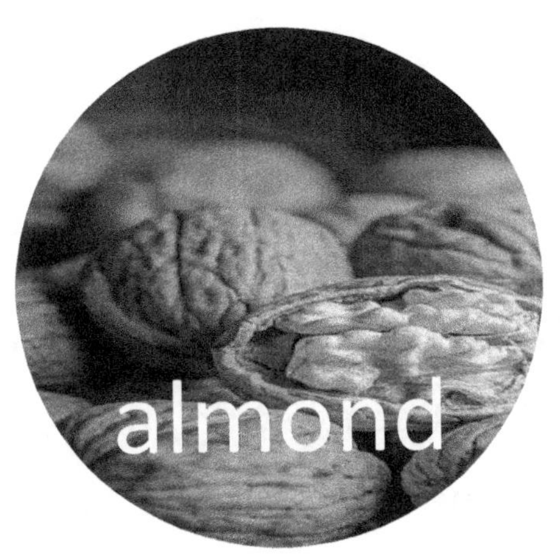

almond

10) Almonds

Almonds are the perfect snack. They are rich in fibre, protein, and heart-healthy fats. They can help you live longer. A study published in The New England Journal of Medicine found that people who ate the most nuts had a lower risk of dying of any disease, particularly cancer, heart disease, or respiratory disease.

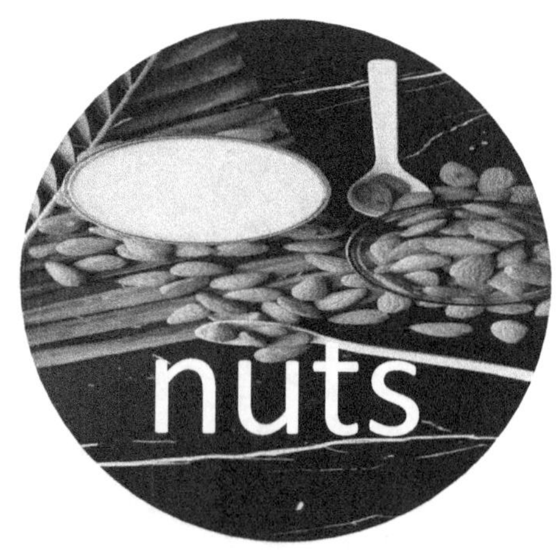

Other important foods are:

- Chia seeds

- Oatmeal

- Bell peppers

- Red wine

- Tomatoes

- Apples

- Coffee

- Dark Chocolate

- Hot peppers

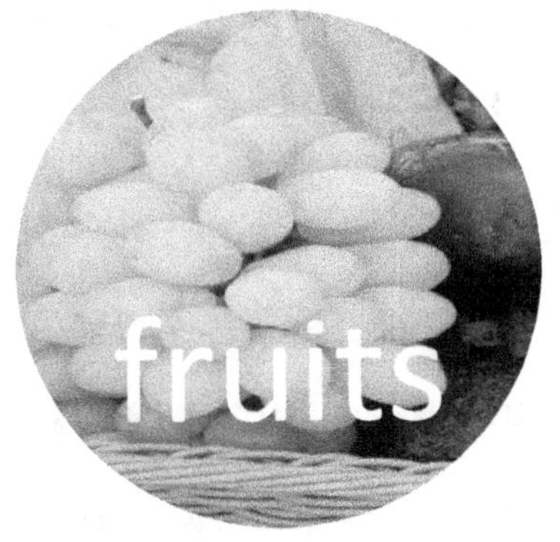

- Yoghurt.

CHAPTER 5

CONCLUSION

Death is inevitable, however, there are still ways we can avoid them. You cannot avoid death but you can make it easier. Practising a healthy lifestyle and eating healthy can go a long way. While none of us will live forever, you can add some extra years to your life by paying special attention to what you eat. What we choose to eat has the potential to help us or harm us. Our addiction to processed food offers inadequate nourishment and is the cause of illnesses like obesity, cardiovascular disease and type 2 diabetes. It shouldn't be this way. It is expected of us to eat foods that leave us energized, reduce our risk of illness and allow us to maintain a healthy weight.

To comfortably live a long and healthy life, we have to fuel our bodies with nutrient-dense foods. Natural plant based foods can replenish our health and vitality.

Asides from eating healthy, regular exercise can help prevent death. Changing certain lifestyle habits such as smoking, taking excess alcohol, taking hard drugs and regular stress can help avoid premature death.